The Ulcer Almanac

Understanding Symptoms, Treating Pain, and Eating Right

Dr Jacob Jabin

TABLE OF CONTENTS

Arterial Ulcers
Symptoms of Arterial Wounds
Causes of Arterial Wounds
Treatment of Arterial Wounds
Treatment of Arterial Wounds
Caring for Arterial Wounds at Home
Foods that may help treat artery ulcers
Recipes for arterial ulcers healing

Venous Ulcer
Venous ulcers formation
Symptoms and Causes
Who does venous ulcers affect
What do venous ulcers look and feel like?
Diagnosis and Tests
Treatments
Arterial vs venous ulcers
Foods that may help treat venous ulcers
Diets

Mouth Ulcers (Canker Sores):
Types of mouth ulcers
Symptoms and Causes
Health issues connected with mouth ulcers
Diagnosis Tests
How to heal mouth ulcers quickly naturally
Prevention
Mouth ulcer vs. canker sore
Foods that may help cure mouth ulcers.

Foods that may help cure mouth ulcers.
Diets

Genital Ulcers
How does this ulcer form
causes
Nonsexually acquired genital ulceration
How genital ulcers look like
Diagnosis and Tests
Management and Treatment
Prevention
Foods that may help treat genital ulcers
Diets

Stomach ulcers
Causes of stomach ulcers
Gastritis
Ulcer or gastritis?
Heartburn
Ulcer pain or heartburn?
Consequences of peptic ulcer
Diagnosis and Tests
Management and Treatment
Surgery (Rare)
Foods that may help cure stomach ulcers
Recipes

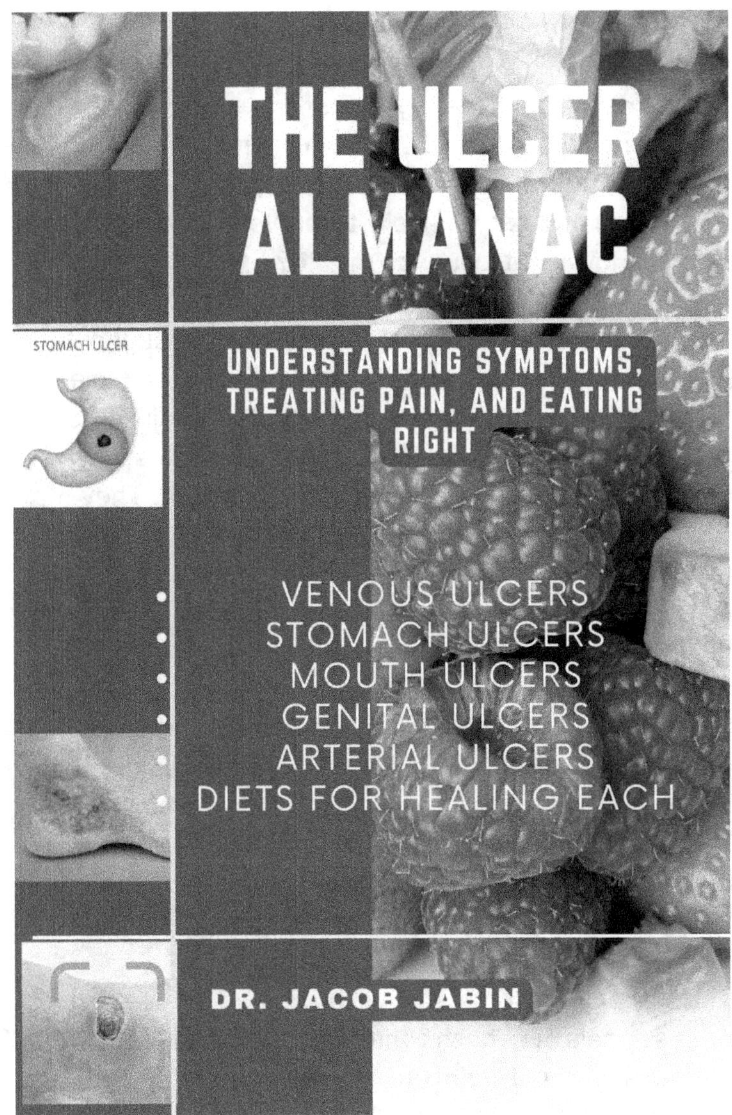

THE ULCER ALMANAC

UNDERSTANDING SYMPTOMS, TREATING PAIN, AND EATING RIGHT

- VENOUS ULCERS
- STOMACH ULCERS
- MOUTH ULCERS
- GENITAL ULCERS
- ARTERIAL ULCERS
- DIETS FOR HEALING EACH

DR. JACOB JABIN

If you are reading this book, chances are you or someone you know has been diagnosed with an ulcer. You may be feeling terrified, bewildered, or overwhelmed by this situation. You may have queries like: What is an ulcer? What causes it? How can I treat it? What can I eat or avoid to prevent it from growing worse? How will it influence my life?

You are not alone. Millions of individuals throughout the globe suffer from ulcers of various forms and places. Ulcers are sores or lesions that occur in the lining of an organ or tissue, such as the stomach, the intestines, the veins, the arteries, the genitals, or the mouth. They may cause discomfort, bleeding, infection, and other consequences. They may also interfere with your everyday activities, your relationships, and your well-being.

But there is hope. Ulcers may be treated and cured with adequate medical treatment and lifestyle adjustments. You may learn how to manage your symptoms, lessen your discomfort, and enhance your quality of life. You may also prevent ulcers from reoccurring or forming in the first place by following some basic suggestions.

That is why we created this book. We are a team of professionals in gastroenterology, vascular surgery, dermatology, and nutrition. We have years of expertise in detecting and treating ulcers of all sorts. We have also witnessed personally how ulcers may influence people's life and how they can overcome them with the correct knowledge and help.

In this book, we will share with you all you need to know about ulcers, from their origins and forms, to their diagnosis and treatment, to their prevention and management. We will also give you with practical suggestions and advise on how to eat correctly, manage with stress, and take care of yourself. We will also address some of the most common and often asked questions concerning ulcers.

Our mission is to help you understand your situation, make educated choices, and take charge of your health. We want you to live a happy and healthy life, free from ulcers.

This book is organized into five segments, each concentrating on a distinct form of ulcer:

- Part One: Arterial Ulcers. These are ulcers that form in the foot or toes, mainly owing to inadequate blood circulation in the arteries. They may induce coldness, numbness, tingling, and gangrene. They may potentially lead to amputation or death.

-Part Two :Venous Ulcers. These are ulcers that form in the lower legs, mainly owing to inadequate blood circulation in the veins. They may cause swelling, discomfort, itching, and skin changes. They may also lead to infections and skin ulcers.

-Part Three : Mouth Ulcers. These are ulcers that form in the mouth, frequently owing to trauma, stress, or immunological problems. They may cause discomfort, trouble eating or speaking, and foul breath. They may also influence your self-esteem and social life.

- Part Four: Genital Ulcers. These are ulcers that arise in the genitals, frequently owing to sexually transmitted illnesses, such as herpes, syphilis, or chancroid. They may cause discomfort, drainage, and enlarged glands. They may also raise the chance of other diseases, such as HIV or HPV.

-Part Five: Mouth Ulcers. These are ulcers that form in the mouth, frequently owing to trauma, stress, or immunological problems. They may cause discomfort, trouble eating or speaking, and foul breath. They may also influence your self-esteem and social life.

-Part Six : Stomach ulcers These are ulcers that arise in the stomach, mainly owing to an infection by a bacteria called Helicobacter pylori, or the use of certain drugs, such as aspirin or ibuprofen. They may induce scorching pain, nausea, vomiting, and bleeding. They may potentially lead to problems like as perforation, blockage, or malignancy.

In each segment, we will describe the causes, symptoms, diagnosis, treatment, and prevention of each form of ulcer. We will also supply you with useful resources and references for additional reading.

We hope that this book will be a great source of knowledge and direction for you and your loved ones. We hope that it will help you deal with your condition and better your position. We hope that it will motivate you to take action and create great changes in your life.

We hope that you will love reading this book as much as we enjoyed creating it. We hope that you will find it helpful and valuable. We hope that you will share it with others who may need help.

We hope that you will cure your ulcers and live your best life.

Arterial Ulcers

Arterial wounds, also known as arterial ulcers, are painful sores in your skin caused by inadequate circulation. Arterial ulcers often form when blood is unable to flow into the lower extremities, such as the legs and feet. When the skin and underlying tissue are deprived of oxygen, the tissue begins to die off and develop an open wound. Arterial wounds tend to be exceedingly painful and unpleasant.

Due to inadequate circulation, arterial wounds may heal slowly. The lack of circulation may also make it harder for the red blood cells to provide the nutrients required to repair. Without oxygen-rich blood, white blood cells might not be able to fight off germs, which will make the wound more prone to get infected. If the wound is left untreated, arterial ulcers may progress to more severe illnesses or consequences, including infection, tissue necrosis, and in extreme circumstances, amputation.

Arterial wounds generally have a punched-out aspect. They may be circular in form with well-defined boundaries implying the sore may be deeper in the skin than the surrounding region of healthy skin.
They're commonly located on the outside ankle, on the heels, on the toes, or in between the toes. They may also arise in regions where there's pressure from walking, exercising, or wearing footwear.

Arterial ulcers also tend to have a particular hue. The wound itself often doesn't bleed and may be black, grey, brown, or yellow. The limb may become crimson when dangling downward, and then pale when held up or lifted.
In addition, you could have:

- There is minimal to no hair development on the affected limb.
- The leg feels chilly to the touch with little to no pulse.
- Your skin and nails looking glossy, thin, and dry
- Your skin feels tight or tense.

Causes of Arterial Wounds

Arterial wounds are most typically caused by obstructed arteries. This may prevent nutrient-rich blood from getting to the extremities, causing an open wound.
Other possible reasons include:

- Poor circulation
- Arteriosclerosis or atherosclerosis
- Venous insufficiency,which is caused by blood in the leg veins not flowing back up to the heart
- Diabetes Kidney failure
- Hypertension (high blood pressure)
- Lying or sitting in one position for too long Other illnesses may also contribute to arterial wounds, including excessive cholesterol, heart disease, high blood pressure, or sickle cell anaemia.

Several risk factors may potentially lead to arterial ulcers, including:

- Diabetes mellitus
- Foot deformity
- Poor footwear Obesity
- Smoking Limited joint mobility

Treatment of Arterial Wounds

Even though your body may repair artery lesions on its own, the natural healing process will be substantially delayed due to circulation difficulties. Many persons with arterial ulcers have persistent discomfort and sores that take months or years to completely cure.

Treatment for arterial ulcers will depend on the severity of the vascular disease. Your physician may undertake diagnostic tests to determine different kinds of therapy, as well as the possibility for wound healing.

Goals for recovery include:

- Improving circulation
- Treating the underlying cause with antibiotics
- Removing touch discomfort and pressure on the affected limb
- Dressing the wound to always keep it dry and clean
- During rehabilitation, you may be required to wear special shoes or orthopaedic equipment to ease pressure on the sore.
- Doctors may employ surgery, including angioplasty, to restore blood flow to tissues in organs. In rare circumstances when blood flow can't be restored, they may propose amputation of the damaged limb.

Caring for Arterial Wounds at Home

Your doctor will give you some guidelines on how to care for your wounds at home. These may include:
- Keeping the wound clean and dry all times by changing the dressing
- Taking all prescription meds
- Drinking lots of water
- Following a healthy diet
- Exercising frequently, as prescribed by your doctor
- Wearing orthopaedic shoes
- Wearing compression wraps if required

To prevent ulcers from forming again or the present ulcers from growing worse there are certain methods you may minimize your risk factor. These include regulating your blood pressure and cholesterol, stopping smoking, exercising frequently (if suitable), and limiting your consumption of salt.

Foods that may help treat artery ulcers

To enhance wound healing, it is necessary to consume a balanced diet that supports your cardiovascular health and decreases inflammation. Some of the foods that may help treat artery ulcers are:

1- **Whole grains:** These are high in fiber, which helps decrease cholesterol and blood pressure, and prevent plaque accumulation in the arteries. Examples of whole grains include brown rice, barley, quinoa, oats, and whole wheat bread.

2- **Legumes:** These are plant-based proteins that also include fiber, antioxidants, and minerals such as calcium, potassium, and magnesium. These nutrients may help decrease blood pressure, enhance blood vessel function, and reduce inflammation. Examples of legumes include beans, lentils, peas, soy, and tofu.

3- **Fatty fish:** These are sources of omega-3 fatty acids, which are anti-inflammatory and help enhance blood flow and avoid blood clots. Omega-3s may help decrease triglycerides and improve healthy cholesterol levels. Examples of fatty fish include salmon, mackerel, tuna, sardines, and herring.

4- **Nuts and seeds:** These are similarly high in omega-3s, as well as fiber, protein, and healthy fats. They may help decrease cholesterol, blood pressure, and inflammation, and protect the blood vessels from injury. Examples of nuts and seeds include walnuts, almonds, pistachios, flaxseeds, chia seeds, and hemp seeds.

5- Fruits and vegetables: These are filled in antioxidants, vitamins, minerals, and phytochemicals that may combat oxidative stress, inflammation, and infection. They may also supply water, fiber, and natural sugars that help keep you hydrated, full, and invigorated. Examples of fruits and vegetables include berries, citrus fruits, apples, bananas, leafy greens, broccoli, carrots, tomatoes, and peppers.

Recipes for arterial ulcers healing

1- Oatmeal with berries and walnuts: Oatmeal is a whole grain that may decrease cholesterol and blood pressure, while berries and walnuts are rich in antioxidants and omega-3s that can reduce inflammation and enhance blood flow. Here is a hint on how to cook oatmeal with berries and walnuts:

- To prepare oatmeal, you will need rolled oats, water, cinnamon, salt, and your choice of berries and walnuts. You may also add some banana, dried fruit, or maple syrup for added sweetness.
- Pour water In a small saucepan, to boil over high heat. Add oats, cinnamon, and salt and decrease the heat to medium-low. Cook until the water is absorbed, approximately 5 to 7 minutes, stirring periodically.
- Stir in some frozen or fresh berries of your choosing. You may use blueberries, raspberries, strawberries, or a blend of them. Top with sliced banana, chopped

walnuts, and/or dried fruit if you desire. Drizzle some maple syrup on top if you want additional sweetness.
- Serve hot and enjoy your tasty and nutritious oatmeal with berries and walnuts.

2- Salmon with quinoa and broccoli: Salmon is a fatty fish that delivers omega-3s, which helps prevent blood clots and protect the blood vessels from damage. Quinoa is another complete grain that provides fiber, protein, and minerals that help improve cardiovascular health. Broccoli is a cruciferous vegetable that contains anti-inflammatory and anti-cancer effects. Salmon with quinoa and broccoli is a nutritious and delightful dinner that you can simply cook at home. Steps to follow:

- Preheat the oven to 200°C (180°C fan) and line a baking pan with parchment paper. Season the salmon fillets with salt, pepper, and some lemon juice and set them on the prepared tray. Bake for 15 to 20 minutes or until the salmon is cooked through and flakes readily with a fork.
- Rinse the quinoa under cold water and drain thoroughly. In a medium saucepan, bring 2 cups of water and a pinch of salt to a boil. Add the quinoa and decrease the heat to low. Cover and boil for 15 to 18 minutes or until the quinoa is frothy and the water is absorbed. Fluff with a fork and keep heated.
- Cut the broccoli into tiny florets and cook them in a steamer basket over boiling water for approximately 10 minutes or until soft but still crisp. You may alternatively

microwave them in a dish with little water for approximately 5 minutes or until done.
- To serve, divide the quinoa among four plates and top with the salmon fillets. Arrange the broccoli on the side and sprinkle some more lemon juice over everything.

3- Bean and vegetable soup: Beans are plant-based proteins that help decrease cholesterol, blood pressure, and inflammation, as well as enhance arterial function and gastrointestinal health. Vegetables including carrots, celery, onion, garlic, and spinach may give antioxidants, vitamins, minerals, and phytochemicals that help combat oxidative stress, infection, and plaque development. Bean and vegetable soup is a substantial and healthy meal that may be created with various components depending on your desire. Here is a generic recipe that you may follow or change as you like:

- Heat some oil in a big saucepan over medium-high heat and sauté some chopped onion, carrot, and celery until tender, approximately 10 minutes. You may also use leek instead of onion for a milder taste.
- Add some minced garlic, salt, pepper, and dried herbs of your choosing, such as thyme, rosemary, or oregano, and simmer for another minute, stirring regularly.
- Stir in some vegetable broth, canned or cooked beans of your choosing, such as white, black, kidney, or chickpeas, and some chopped tomatoes, fresh or canned. You may also add some additional veggies,

such as zucchini, green beans, broccoli, or spinach, if you prefer.
- Bring the soup to a boil, then decrease the heat and simmer until the beans and veggies are cooked, approximately 20 to 30 minutes. You may also mash some of the beans with a potato masher or a fork to thicken the soup if you want.
- Taste and adjust the seasoning as required. Serve hot with some bread, crackers, or croutons, and enjoy!

4- Tofu and vegetable stir-fry: Tofu is a complete soy food that helps decrease cholesterol, blood pressure, and triglycerides, as well as enhance blood vessel function and reduce inflammation. Vegetables like bell peppers, mushrooms, zucchini, and bok choy may give fiber, water, and natural sugars that help keep you hydrated, full, and invigorated. Tofu and vegetable stir-fry is a simple and tasty recipe that you may prepare with various components. Some steps to follow:

- Cut the tofu into tiny cubes and press them with a paper towel to remove excess water. Season them with salt, pepper, and little cornstarch.
- Heat some oil in a big pan or wok over high heat and cook the tofu until brown and crisp on both sides. Transfer to a platter and keep heated.
- In the same pan, add some additional oil and stir-fry your choice of veggies until crisp-tender. You may use broccoli, carrots, bell peppers, mushrooms, snap peas, or any other vegetables you choose.

- In a small bowl, mix together some soy sauce, vegetable broth, honey, sesame oil, garlic, ginger, and cornstarch to produce a sauce. Pour the sauce over the veggies and bring to a boil. Cook until the sauce is thickened, stirring periodically.
- Add the tofu back to the pan and stir to coat with the sauce. Sprinkle some sesame seeds and sliced scallions on top if desired.
- Serve hot over rice, noodles, or quinoa and enjoy your tofu and veggie stir-fry.

5- Avocado and tomato salad: Avocado is a fruit that provides healthy fats, fiber, and antioxidants that help decrease cholesterol, blood pressure, and inflammation, as well as enhance blood vessel function and protect against cellular damage. Tomato is another food that includes lycopene, a potent antioxidant that helps reduce oxidative stress and plaque development. Avocado and tomato salad is a fresh and colorful side dish that can be produced with a few basic ingredients. Here is a potential note on how to prepare it:

- In a separate bowl, mix together 1/4 cup of extra-virgin olive oil, the juice of 1 lemon, 1/4 teaspoon of ground cumin, salt, and pepper to produce a dressing.
- In a large bowl, mix together 3 cubed avocados, 1 pint of halved cherry tomatoes, 1 sliced cucumber, 1/3 cup of corn, 1 minced jalapeño (optional), and 2 tablespoons of chopped cilantro.
- Drizzle the dressing over the salad and gently stir to blend.

- You can serve immediately or refrigerate until ready to eat.

6- Green tea with dark chocolate: Green tea is a beverage that includes catechins, antioxidants that help increase blood flow and prevent blood clots. Dark chocolate is a treat that contains flavonoids, antioxidants that can lower blood pressure, improve blood vessel function, and reduce inflammation. Green tea and dark chocolate are both tasty and nutritious delights that may be enjoyed together. Here are some alternative methods to prepare them:

- You may create green tea chocolate by melting white chocolate and combining it with cream, butter, and matcha powder. Then you can pour the mixture into a form and chill it until hard. Cut into little pieces and sprinkle with extra matcha powder if you want.
- You may create matcha dark chocolate truffles by boiling milk and pouring it over chopped dark chocolate. Whisk until smooth and add with some matcha powder. Refrigerate the ingredients until hard and then form into balls. You may cover them with cocoa powder, almonds, or additional matcha powder.
- You may create a simple green tea and dark chocolate combo by making some green tea of your choosing and serving it with a few pieces of dark chocolate. You may experiment with several varieties of green tea, such as sencha, gyokuro, jasmine, or genmaicha, and see how they enhance the taste of the chocolate.

Venous Ulcer

Venous leg ulcers are persistent lesions on the lower leg produced by inadequate venous return from the foot to the heart (due to varicose or obstructed veins). They mainly afflict elderly individuals, with some estimates indicating up to 1% of persons will be affected by a leg ulcer at some time in their lives in industrialized nations with greater frequency in females aged over 70 years . The average cost of treating a venous ulcer with dressings ranged between €1332 and €2585 in Sweden and from €814 to €1994 in the United Kingdom (UK) . The cost-of-illness of leg ulcer therapy in Hamburg found mean yearly total expenses of €9060/patient/year and related high costs of leg ulcers for health insurances, patients and society . The incidence in less industrialised nations is not thoroughly reported as yet, although it is probable that venous ulcers may also affect individuals across contexts. Leg ulcers generally take months to cure fully and frequently return after healing. Some individuals are troubled with venous ulcers for many years and the loss of wound fluid from the ulcer, stench, irritation and discomfort may diminish quality of life and self image, and sometimes lead to poor mood and despair .

Venous ulcers are lesions that take weeks, or occasionally months, to cure. They may deteriorate fast, placing you at risk for complications that lead some individuals to lose their limbs. With good therapy, you may prevent these complications.

Venous ulcers formation

Venous ulcers form when oxygen-poor blood can't travel from your extremities back to your heart. Instead, it pools, generating pressure in your veins. This affects skin tissue and leads to an ulcer.

Symptoms and Causes

What causes venous ulcers?
Your veins have microscopic valves that keep blood moving throughout your body. These valves snap open and close to flow blood against the force of gravity back to your heart. In certain cases, venous disorders compromise valve functionality. Other medical disorders, including diabetes, might also put you at risk for leg and foot ulcers.

What forms of venous illness create venous stasis ulcers?

Chronic venous insufficiency is a frequent cause of valve malfunction. It happens when your valves are broken or too weak to complete their function.

Other venous ulcer causes include:

- High blood pressure (hypertension), which destroys blood vessel walls.
- Venous obstruction, a vein blockage that's occasionally linked to blood clots.
- Venous reflux, when blood flows backward via weak or broken valves.

Who does venous ulcers affect

A lot of factors might boost your risk of venous ulcers. They include:

- Deep vein thrombosis.
- Family history of venous illness.
- Obesity.
- Older age.
- Paralysis.
- Previous injury.
- Sedentary lifestyle with minimal physical exercise.
- Smoking.
- Surgery, such as a knee replacement.
- Varicose and spider veins.

What do venous ulcers look and feel like?

They're frequently shallow, oddly formed lesions. The skin around the stasis ulcer may be firm and pigmented.

Symptoms of venous ulcers include

- Dull pain.
- Foul odor.
- Itching.
- Pus or other fluid that pours from the sore.
- Swelling (edema)

Diagnosis and Tests

Venous stasis ulcers are identified using a combination of clinical examination and specialized testing. Let's go into the details:

1. Clinical Examination:
- Physical examination plays a significant role in identifying venous stasis ulcers. Here's what healthcare experts look for:
  - Appearance of the Ulcer: Venous ulcers are often uneven and shallow with well-defined

boundaries. They commonly arise above bony prominences.

- Skin Changes: Look for symptoms of venous illness, such as varicose veins, edema, or venous dermatitis.

Other Associated Findings may include telangiectasias, corona phlebectatica, atrophie blanche, lipodermatosclerosis, and the inverted champagne-bottle deformity of the lower leg.

2. Specific Tests:

- Ankle-Brachial Index (ABI): This test monitors blood pressure in your arms and legs. It helps measure blood flow and diagnose arterial occlusive disease.

- Doppler research: By listening to blood flow via your veins, this research examines venous circulation.

- Imaging Studies: Techniques like CT scans may reveal damaged or non functioning valves in the veins.

3. Duplex Ultrasound:

- This imaging examination offers extensive information about blood flow and the anatomy of leg veins. It examines the speed and direction of blood flow in the blood vessels.

Venous ulcers don't cure on their own. The longer you live with them, the higher the potential of lasting tissue damage. The damage may spread or produce infections that can become life- or limb-threatening, such as gangrene.

In extreme circumstances, it may be required to surgically remove (amputate) your damaged limb. Timely treatment from a skilled wound care clinician considerably minimizes this risk.

Treatments

Venous leg ulcers may be tough, but with adequate treatment, they commonly recover within 6 months. It's necessary to engage with a healthcare expert skilled in compression treatment for leg ulcers. Here are some significant treatments:

1. Cleaning and Dressing the Ulcer:
- The first step entails removing debris or dead tissue from the ulcer, cleaning and drying it, and putting a suitable dressing. This generates perfect circumstances for healing.
- A basic non-sticky dressing is commonly used and has to be changed 1 to 3 times a week.
- Many people can manage to clean and dress their own ulcer when a nurse supervises them .

2. Compression:
- To improve vein circulation and reduce swelling, a firm compression bandage is applied over the affected leg.

- These bandages encourage blood flow upward toward the heart.
- Compression bandages are usually changed 1 to 3 times a week during dressing changes.
- Initially, applying compression bandages may cause discomfort, but the pain lessens as the ulcer heals.
- If the bandage feels too tight or uncomfortable at night, a short walk can help. However, if you experience numbness, tingling, unusual pain, or swelling, seek medical attention promptly.

3- Exercise: Regular physical activity, especially exercises that engage the calf muscles, can enhance blood circulation and aid in healing venous ulcers.

4- Medications:
Pentoxifylline: This medication can improve blood flow and may be prescribed to enhance healing.

Growth Factor Therapy: Injectable substances that attract healthy cells to the ulcers.

Hyperbaric Oxygen Therapy: In this treatment, you sit in a special, pressurized chamber and inhale pure oxygen.

Lymphedema Therapy: This includes massage, skin care, and bandaging techniques to clear fluid buildup.

5- Referral to a Wound Specialist: Consider contacting a wound subspecialist if your ulcers are big, of protracted duration, or recalcitrant to conservative therapy.

Arterial vs venous ulcers

These frequent lower extremity wounds may be challenging to recognize, since they have numerous similarities. However, several crucial qualities can help you accurately identify them.

Let's investigate the distinctions between venous ulcers and arterial or ischemic ulcers. Knowing their major aspects, such as location and size, may help you decide optimal wound management and enhance patient outcomes.

Arterial Ulcers

Location: Arterial ulcers, caused by a lack of blood circulation, mostly occur often on the foot, at the tips of the toes or in between, at areas that has pressure from foot wear, around lateral malleolus (the bone on the outside of the ankle joint) and on the heels.

Size and shape: Most typically round, with a "punched out" appearance, they may range in size from microscopic to large, with well-defined edges.

Color: Often seems yellow, brown or black in color. Skin may also look pale and non-granulating.

Appearance: Arterial ulcers are generally deep, although may occasionally look shallow in early stages. Skin surrounding the wound is typically thin, smooth, tight and dry. Loss of hair on the leg is also prevalent.

Exudate: Unlike venous ulcers, artery ulcers are often dry due to limited drainage.

Pain level: Reportedly pretty intense. Elevating the leg could increase this soreness.

Other unique characteristics:

- Toenails often look brittle, yellow, malformed, thick and dry.
- A patient's pulse may be discernible around the location of the incision.
- The region surrounding the incision is likely chilly or icy to the touch owing to insufficient blood circulation.

Venous Ulcers

Location: Venous leg ulcers commonly occur on the inner lower leg, above the medial malleolus, gaiter region.

Size and shape: Wounds are frequently shallow, yet big, and often have uneven margins that may also slope.

Color: Typically, venous wounds look reddish red, with granular tissue. There may also be discolouration with yellow slough present.

Appearance: Surrounding skin may be glossy, heated or scaly. Tunnelling is unusual.

Exudate: These wounds generally seem moist, since they often contain moderate to heavy exudate, needing absorbent wound care coverings.

Other information and advice concerning venous ulcers:

- When it gets infected, there is mostly an accompanying foul odor, and may be purulent.
- Venous ulcers are the most frequent kind of lower extremity lesion, accounting for 80% to 90% of all leg ulcers.
- Venous leg ulcers commonly return. That's why it's vital to treat the underlying venous sickness with compression and other therapies.

Foods that may help treat venous ulcers

Venous ulcers are lesions that arise owing to inadequate blood flow to the legs and feet. They may be painful, sluggish to heal, and prone to infection. To enhance wound healing, it is necessary to consume a balanced diet that promotes your vascular health and lowers inflammation. Some of the foods that may help treat venous ulcers are:

- **Lean meats:** These are sources of protein, which is needed for tissue regeneration and wound healing. Lean meats like skinless chicken and lean beef may also contain iron, zinc, and vitamin B12, which are crucial for blood formation and oxygen transport. Avoid processed meats, such as bacon, ham, and sausages, since they might raise inflammation and blood pressure.

- **Fish and seafood:** These are also high in protein and omega-3 fatty acids, which are anti-inflammatory and help enhance blood flow and prevent blood clots. Fish and seafood may also supply iodine, selenium, and vitamin D, which are crucial for thyroid function and immune system health.

- **Eggs:** These are another source of protein and omega-3s, as well as biotin, a vitamin that may aid with skin health and wound healing. Eggs may also supply choline, a substance that can aid with neuron function and muscular contraction.

- **Whole soy foods:** These are plant-based proteins that help decrease cholesterol, blood pressure, and inflammation, as well as enhance blood vessel function and reduce oxidative stress. Whole soy foods like tofu or tempeh may also include calcium, magnesium, and phytoestrogens, which can aid with bone health and hormone balance.

- **Fermented dairy foods:** These are sources of probiotics, helpful microorganisms that may aid with gut health and immune system function. Fermented dairy foods like kefir or yogurt may also supply protein, calcium, and vitamin K2, which can aid with blood coagulation and bone health .

- **Healthy fats:** These are fats that help decrease cholesterol, blood pressure, and inflammation, as well as enhance blood vessel function and protect against cellular damage. Healthy fats like olive oil, avocados, and almonds may also supply vitamin E, a potent antioxidant that can aid with skin health and wound healing .

- **Whole and cracked grains:** These are grains that have not been refined or treated, and contain their bran, germ, and endosperm. Whole and broken grains may contain fiber, which helps decrease cholesterol and blood pressure, and avoid constipation and infection. They may also contain B vitamins, iron, magnesium, and phytochemicals, which can aid with energy generation and blood formation .

- **Green tea:** This is a beverage that includes catechins, antioxidants that help increase blood flow and prevent blood clots. Green tea may also include caffeine, which can aid with alertness and mood .

Diets

Diets that may help treat venous ulcers and how to prepare them. Here are several examples:

1- Lean turkey and veggie wrap: Lean turkey is a source of protein, which is needed for wound healing. It also offers iron, zinc, and vitamin B12, which are needed for blood formation and oxygen transport. Vegetables like lettuce, tomato, and cucumber may give antioxidants, vitamins, minerals, and phytochemicals that help combat infection and inflammation. A lean turkey and veggie wrap is a simple and nutritious lunch that you can cook with a few ingredients. Here is a potential note on how to prepare it:

- You will need a tortilla, some hummus, some sliced turkey, and some chopped veggies of your choosing. You may use lettuce, tomato, cucumber, bell pepper, or any other vegetables you choose.
- Lay the tortilla on a flat surface and spread some hummus over it. Leave some room around the borders.
- Arrange the turkey slices on top of the hummus, covering roughly half of the tortilla.
- Sprinkle the chopped veggies over the turkey, adding as much or as little as you desire.

- Fold the bottom edge of the tortilla over the filling, then fold in the sides and roll up the tortilla from the bottom to the top. Cut the wrap in half and you are good to go.

2- Fish and seafood stew: Fish and seafood are rich in protein and omega-3 fatty acids, which are anti-inflammatory and help enhance blood flow and prevent blood clots. They also include iodine, selenium, and vitamin D, which are crucial for thyroid function and immune system health. Fish and seafood stew is a wonderful and substantial meal that may be created with many types of seafood, such as clams, mussels, shrimp, scallops, and white fish. Here is a potential note on how to prepare it:

- In a large saucepan, heat some olive oil over medium-high heat and sauté some chopped onion, garlic, fennel, and red pepper flakes until tender, approximately 10 minutes.
- Stir in some tomato paste, white wine, fish or vegetable broth, bay leaf, and salt and pepper and bring the stew to a boil. Reduce the heat and simmer for 15 minutes.
- Add the clams and mussels and simmer until they open, removing any that do not open, around 10 minutes.
- Add the shrimp, scallops, and white fish and cook until they are opaque and cooked through, approximately 5 minutes.

- Stir in some chopped parsley and serve the stew with crusty bread or rice.

3- Egg and spinach scramble: Eggs are another source of protein and omega-3s, as well as biotin, a vitamin that may aid with skin health and wound healing. They also include choline, a vitamin that may aid with neuron function and muscular contraction. Spinach is a leafy green food that may deliver antioxidants, vitamins, minerals, and phytochemicals that help combat oxidative stress, infection, and plaque development. Egg and spinach scramble is a simple and nutritious meal that you can cook using eggs, spinach, onion, garlic, salt, pepper, and cheese. Here is a potential note on how to prepare it:

- In a small bowl, mix four eggs with a sprinkle of salt and pepper and 1/4 cup of shredded cheese. You may use whatever cheese you desire, such as cheddar, mozzarella, or parmesan.
- In a large pan, heat some oil over medium-high heat and sauté one sliced onion until tender, approximately 10 minutes. Add two minced garlic cloves and simmer for another minute, stirring constantly.
- Add four cups of fresh spinach leaves and simmer until wilted, approximately 5 minutes. You may also use frozen spinach, but be sure to defrost and strain out the extra water first.
- Reduce the heat to medium-low and pour the egg mixture over the spinach. Stir gently to incorporate and

heat until the eggs are set, approximately 10 minutes. You may also cover the skillet with a lid to speed up the cooking process.
- Serve hot with some bread, toast, or fruit.

4- Tofu and vegetable curry: Tofu is a complete soy food that helps decrease cholesterol, blood pressure, and inflammation, as well as enhance blood vessel function and minimize oxidative stress. It also includes calcium, magnesium, and phytoestrogens, which may aid with bone health and hormonal balance. Vegetables like cauliflower, potato, and peas may give fiber, water, and natural sugars that help keep you hydrated, satisfied, and invigorated. Tofu and vegetable curry is a wonderful and substantial meal that may be cooked using numerous types of vegetables, such as carrots, peas, spinach, and tomatoes. Here is a potential note on how to prepare it:

- Cut the tofu into little chunks and mix them with some cornstarch, salt, pepper, and garam masala. Fry them in some oil till brown and crisp on both sides. Set aside.
- In the same pan, heat some additional oil and sauté some chopped onion and ginger until tender. Add some tomato paste, garlic, curry powder, cumin, coriander, turmeric, and cayenne and simmer for a few minutes, stirring regularly.
- Stir in some vegetable broth and coconut milk and bring the sauce to a boil. Reduce the heat and simmer for approximately 15 minutes, until slightly thickened.

- Add the veggies of your choosing and simmer until soft, around 10 to 15 minutes. You may use fresh or frozen veggies, such as carrots, peas, spinach, and tomatoes.
- Stir in the tofu and some chopped cilantro and season with salt and pepper to taste.
- Serve hot with rice, naan bread, or roti and enjoy your tofu and veggie curry.

5- Avocado and tomato toast: Avocado is a fruit that provides healthy fats, fiber, and antioxidants that help decrease cholesterol, blood pressure, and inflammation, as well as enhance blood vessel function and protect against cellular damage. It also includes vitamin E, a potent antioxidant that may aid with skin health and wound healing. Tomato is another food that includes lycopene, a potent antioxidant that helps reduce oxidative stress and plaque development. Avocado and tomato toast is a simple and tasty food that you can create using bread, avocado, tomato, lemon juice, salt, pepper, and maybe some cheese, garlic, balsamic vinegar, and olive oil. Here are some probable actions to follow:

- Toast your bread until it's brown and crunchy. You may use whatever sort of bread you choose, such as whole wheat, sourdough, or baguette.
- Cut one avocado in half and remove the pit. Scoop out the meat and mash it with a fork in a small basin.

Squeeze some lemon juice over the avocado and season with salt and pepper to taste.
- Spread the avocado mixture equally over the bread pieces. You may also add some cheese, such as feta, mozzarella, or parmesan, if you prefer.
- Slice a tomato and lay it on top of the avocado toast. You may also add some garlic, balsamic vinegar, and olive oil for extra taste.
- Enjoy your avocado and tomato toast as a breakfast, snack, or light meal.

6- Green tea with dark chocolate: Green tea is a beverage that includes catechins, antioxidants that help increase blood flow and prevent blood clots. It also includes caffeine, which may aid with alertness and mood. Dark chocolate is a delicacy that includes flavonoids, antioxidants that help decrease blood pressure, enhance blood vessel function, and reduce inflammation.Green tea and dark chocolate are both tasty and healthful treats that can be enjoyed together. Here are some alternative methods to prepare them:

- You may create green tea chocolate by melting white chocolate and combining it with cream, butter, and matcha powder. Then you can pour the mixture into a form and chill it until hard. Cut into little pieces and sprinkle with extra matcha powder if you want.
- You may create matcha dark chocolate truffles by boiling milk and pouring it over chopped dark chocolate. Whisk until smooth and add with some matcha powder.

Refrigerate the ingredients until hard and then form into balls. You may cover them with cocoa powder, almonds, or additional matcha powder.
- You may create a simple green tea and dark chocolate combo by making some green tea of your choosing and serving it with a few pieces of dark chocolate. You may experiment with several varieties of green tea, such as sencha, gyokuro, jasmine, or genmaicha, and see how they enhance the taste of the chocolate.

Mouth Ulcers (Canker Sores):

A mouth ulcer is a sore that occurs anywhere within your mouth. These sores are generally red, yellow or white, and you can have one or numerous.

You may acquire mouth ulcers on your:

- Gums.
- Tongue.
- Roof of mouth (palate).
- Inner cheeks.
- Inner lips.

These sores are sometimes unpleasant and may make eating, drinking and speaking difficult.

Mouth ulcers may be scary. However, they're not a sexually transmitted illness (STI) and you can't catch or spread them by kissing or sharing food and beverages. Aside from any pain and discomfort, mouth ulcers are usually harmless and go away on their own in a week or two. Some types of mouth sores could point to underlying health conditions like viruses, gastrointestinal issues or autoimmune diseases

Types of mouth ulcers

There are numerous distinct forms of mouth sores and lesions, including:

1- Canker sores (aphthous ulcers). These are the most prevalent form of mouth ulcers. Healthcare experts aren't precisely clear what causes them or why some individuals get them more than others do. Causes include acidic foods ,minor trauma (like biting your cheek) and even stress. Canker sores are generally white or yellow with red around the borders.

2- Oral lichen planus. This illness may produce itchy rashes and lacelike, white lesions within your mouth. Oral lichen planus is known as an immune system response and most commonly affects people assigned female at birth (AFAB) age 50 or older and women.

3- Leukoplakia. Leukoplakia causes grey or white patches inside your mouth. It develops because of excess cell growth. Chronic inflammation from things like smoking or chewing tobacco might cause it. It does happens sometimes for no apparent reason. Leukoplakia lesions normally aren't malignant.

4- Erythroplakia. This is another symptom of chewing tobacco or smoking. People with this have red patches that normally appear behind their lower front teeth or under their tongue. Compared to leukoplakia lesions, erythroplakia patches are mostly precancerous or cancerous.

5- Oral thrush. An excess of yeast called Candida albicans causes this fungal illness within your mouth. It typically occurs after antibiotic treatment or when your immune system isn't as robust as it normally is. Oral thrush creates red and creamy white mouth sores and patches.

6- Mouth cancer. Oral cancer lesions could show up as white or red mouth sores or ulcers. These lesions won't cure on their own. If you develop a mouth ulcer that hasn't gone away after three weeks, inform your healthcare provider

Symptoms and Causes

What are the signs of a mouth ulcer?
Mouth ulcers are typically simple to notice. They show as sores on your gums, tongue, inner cheeks, inner lips or roof of your mouth.

Mouth sores are typically:

- Red across the borders.
- White, yellow or gray in the middle.

You may just get one ulcer, or there may be several. Other symptoms might include:

- Swelling around the ulcers.
- Increased pain while cleaning your teeth.
- Pain that intensifies with eating spicy, salty or sour foods

Causes of mouth ulcers

Mouth ulcers may arise for a variety of causes, including:

- Minor tissue harm from dental procedure, such as having a cavity filled.
- Accidentally biting your face or tongue.
- An allergic response to specific germs.
- Wearing braces or retainers.
- Using strong or abrasive toothpaste.
- Eating plenty of acidic foods, such as oranges, pineapples and strawberries.
- Hormonal changes throughout your period.
- Stress.
- Lack of sleep.

Health issues connected with mouth ulcers

Certain health disorders, including numerous autoimmune illnesses, may also induce mouth ulcers. These conditions may include:

- Vitamin deficiency.
- Viral, bacterial or fungal infections.
- Crohn's disease.
- Celiac illness.

Diagnosis Tests

A healthcare professional may detect a mouth ulcer with a visual examination. If you have a serious breakout, or if they suspect a particular health concern, they may prescribe blood testing.

Management and Treatment
How do you cure a mouth ulcer?
While most mouth sores heal on their own, your physician may prescribe drugs to assist alleviate pain. Common mouth ulcer treatments include:

- Antiseptic gels or mouth rinses like (Orajel™) or (Anbesol®).
- Steroid ointments like triamcinolone.
- Immunosuppressants (in extreme situations).

How to heal mouth ulcers quickly naturally

There are various things you may do at home to ease mouth sore symptoms:

- Drink lots of water.
- Practice proper oral hygiene to keep your mouth as clean as possible.
- Try to rinse your mouth with warm saltwater a few times a day.
- Make a combination of equal parts hydrogen peroxide and water and rinse your mouth twice a day.
- Avoid hot and spicy meals until the ulcer heals.
- Use (OTC) topical anesthetic like (Orajel™) or (Anbesol®) which are over-the-counter

Prevention

While you can't avoid mouth ulcers totally, there are things you can do to lower your risk:

- Brush your teeth twice daily and floss once everyday for excellent oral health.
- Use a soft-bristled toothbrush to prevent tissue irritation.
- Eat a nutritious diet rich in fresh fruits and vegetables.
- Visit your dentist periodically for exams and cleanings.

How long do mouth ulcers last?

In most situations, mouth ulcers go away on their own in approximately 10 to 14 days. If you have a mouth sore that lasts longer than three weeks, arrange an appointment with your healthcare practitioner.

Contact your healthcare professional in case of :

- Mouth sores that linger for three weeks or more.
- New sores that emerge before the existing ones heal.
- Mouth ulcers that damage the outside region of your lips.
- Pain that doesn't improve with medicine.
- Unusually huge mouth ulcers.
- Mouth sores that are painless.
- Fever.
- Diarrhea.

Mouth ulcer vs. canker sore

Mouth ulcer is a comprehensive word that defines any pain or lesion within your mouth. As we discussed previously, canker sores are the most frequent kind of oral ulcer. They impact around 20% of the overall population. Many individuals use the words mouth ulcer and canker sore interchangeably.

You could acquire a canker sore if you have a folate, vitamin B or iron deficit. But in most situations, canker sores arise without a recognized origin and for no obvious reason. They may also recur (return), meaning they come and go throughout the course of your lifetime.

Foods that may help cure mouth ulcers.

While most mouth ulcers heal on their own within a week or two, there are many foods that may help speed up the healing process and minimize the discomfort. These foods include:

- **Vitamin B-rich foods:** Vitamin B is necessary for the health of your mouth and skin, and a lack of it may contribute to mouth ulcers. Some great sources of vitamin B are fish, eggs, tofu, dairy products, shellfish, and whole grains.

- **Iron-rich foods:** Iron helps your body generate red blood cells, which supply oxygen to your tissues and promote healing. Iron deficiency may also cause mouth ulcers, so make sure you consume enough iron-rich foods, such as beef, poultry, fish, beans, spinach, broccoli, and dried fruits.

- **Fruits:** Fruits are rich in vitamin C, which is a strong antioxidant that helps enhance your immune system and fight infections. Vitamin C may also help prevent and cure mouth ulcers by promoting collagen synthesis and tissue repair. Some fruits that are high in vitamin C include citrus fruits, kiwi, berries, and papaya.

- Honey: Honey is a natural sweetener that contains antibacterial, anti-inflammatory, and wound-healing characteristics. It may help ease the pain and inflammation of oral ulcers, as well as prevent infection and speed up healing. You may apply honey directly to your mouth ulcers after each meal, or blend it with warm water and ingest it.

- Coconut products: Coconut oil, water, and milk are all good for mouth ulcers, as they include anti-inflammatory, antibacterial, and moisturizing effects. They may help lessen the swelling and pain of mouth ulcers, as well as protect them from drying up and splitting. You may swish coconut oil or water in your mouth, or ingest coconut milk to gain the benefits.

Diets

six meals that may help heal mouth ulcers that are very easy to swallow or chew without hurting your sore mouth. These are how to prepare them. Here you go:

1- Egg salad sandwich: An egg salad sandwich is a simple and appetizing meal that you can create with just a few ingredients. Here are the key procedures to construct an egg salad sandwich:

- Boil 8 eggs in a pot of water for 10 minutes, then drain and chill them in cold water.
- Peel the eggs and slice them into tiny pieces. You now transfer them to a bowl and mash them with a fork.
- Add 1/2 cup of mayonnaise, salt and pepper to taste, and any other flavors you desire, such as mustard, lemon juice, celery, onion, or pickle relish. Mix well to mix.
- Spoon the egg salad over your choice of bread, such as rolls, croissants, or sliced bread. You may also add lettuce, tomato, avocado, or bacon for extra flavor and texture.
- Enjoy your egg salad sandwich or keep it in the refrigerator for up to 5 days.

2- Yoghurt parfait: A yogurt parfait is a healthy and delightful meal that you can create using yogurt, granola, and fresh fruits. Here are some simple strategies to build a yogurt parfait:

- Choose your favorite yogurt, such as plain, vanilla, or Greek style. You may also add additional honey, maple syrup, or vanilla essence to sweeten it if you want.
- Choose your favorite granola, such as homemade, store-bought, or muesli. You may also add some nuts, seeds, or dried fruits for extra crunch and minerals.

- Choose your favorite fruits, such as berries, bananas, apples, peaches, or mangoes. You may also use canned or frozen fruits if fresh ones are not available.
- Layer the yogurt, granola, and fruits in a clear glass or a jar. You may start with yogurt, then granola, then fruits, or any order you like. You now repeat the layers until the glass or jar is full.
- Enjoy your yogurt parfait right now or refrigerate it for later. You may also top it with some whipped cream, chocolate, or nut butter for a more sumptuous dessert.

3- Banana smoothie: A banana smoothie is a delightful and healthful drink that you can produce with just a few ingredients. This is a simple recipe for a banana smoothie:

- Peel and slice a banana and put it into a blender. For a thicker and colder smoothie, add a frozen banana.
- Add 1 cup of milk and 1/4 cup of plain or vanilla yogurt. You may also use almond milk, soy milk, or coconut milk for a dairy-free version.
- Add 1 teaspoon of honey, maple syrup, or vanilla essence for some sweetness. You may also add extra cinnamon, nutmeg, or cocoa powder for enhanced flavor.
- Blend everything until smooth and creamy. In case the smoothie is too thick, add additional milk. If it is too thin, add extra ice cubes or more bananas.

- Pour the smoothie into a glass and enjoy. You may also top it with some banana slices, whipped cream, or granola.

This dish is a soft and easy-to-eat fruit that may treat your mouth ulcers. It is rich in potassium, magnesium, and vitamin C, which aids in enhancing healing and lowering inflammation.

4- Chicken noodle soup: Here is a guideline on how to create chicken noodle soup

- Pat chicken dry with paper towels; sprinkle with salt and pepper. In a saucepan, heat oil over medium-high heat. Add chicken in batches, cook until golden brown, about 5 minutes. Remove chicken from pot; remove all but 2 tablespoons of drippings.

- Add onion and celery to drippings; cook and stir until tender, about 5 minutes. Add garlic; cook 1 minute longer. Add chicken stock and vegetable broth, stirring to remove browned chunks from the pot. Bring to a boil. Return chicken to pot. Add carrots, bay leaves, and thyme. Reduce heat; simmer, covered, until chicken is cooked through, about 25 minutes.

- Transfer chicken to a plate. Remove soup from heat. Add noodles; let rest, covered, until noodles are soft, about 20 minutes. Meanwhile, when chicken is cool enough to handle, pull meat from bones; discard bones. Shred meat into bite-sized pieces. Return meat to pot. Stir in parsley and lemon juice. Season with salt and pepper to taste. Discard bay leaves.

- Enjoy your chicken noodle soup!

It is very easy to ingest and does not worsen your mouth ulcers.

5- Macaroni and cheese:

- Cook the macaroni in a large pot of boiling salted water until al dente, about 8 to 10 minutes. Drain and transfer to a 9x13 inch baking dish.
- In a medium skillet over medium heat, melt 6 tablespoons of butter and whisk in 6 teaspoons of flour. Cook for 2 minutes, stirring frequently, to form a roux.
- Gradually whisk in 4 cups of milk and bring the sauce to a boil. Reduce the heat and simmer, stirring periodically, until slightly thickened, approximately 10 minutes.
- Stir in 4 cups of shredded cheddar cheese, cheese, 1/4 cup of grated parmesan ,1 teaspoon of salt, and 1/4 teaspoon of black pepper. Cook and whisk until the cheese is melted and the sauce is smooth.
- Pour the cheese sauce over the macaroni and swirl to coat completely. Sprinkle 1/4 cup of breadcrumbs and 2 tablespoons of melted butter over the top.
- Bake the macaroni and cheese in a preheated oven at 350°F for 30 minutes, or until the topping is golden and bubbly.
- Enjoy your homemade macaroni and cheese! You may also add some cooked bacon, ham, chicken, or veggies for added taste and texture.

6- Pudding: Pudding is a baked, sweet dish with a soft, creamy, silky feel. It often comprises milk or cream,

sugar, cornstarch, and flavorings such as vanilla, chocolate, or fruit.

- To prepare pudding, you need to put the sugar, cornstarch, and salt in a pot, then gently whisk in the milk. Bring the mixture to a boil over medium heat, stirring frequently, until it thickens. Cook for a few more minutes, then remove from the heat and whisk in the flavorings.

- You may also add eggs to the pudding for a richer and smoother texture. To achieve this, you need to whisk the egg yolks in a small bowl, then gradually whisk in portions of the heated milk mixture. Then, add the egg mixture to the pot and simmer until thickened, stirring constantly.

- Pour the hot pudding into dessert cups or moulds that have been washed in cold water. Cover with plastic wrap and refrigerate until hard, at least 2 hours. Enjoy your pudding as it is, or with whipped cream, nuts, or fruit toppings.

Genital Ulcers

An ulcer is a slow-healing sore. It often occurs along your digestive system, including your stomach. But ulcers may also grow in your vaginal region on the:

- Anus.
- Outer section of your vagina (vulva).
- Penis.
- Skin near these locations

How does this ulcer form

Ulcers frequently arise owing to viruses, bacteria and germs that irritate the genitals' delicate tissue. The body reacts by releasing specific cells that aggravate the discomfort. This causes tiny sores to grow. Once you have an ulcer, continual bacteria exposure makes it harder for the ulcer to heal. Anyone may have genital ulcers. Sexually transmitted infections (STIs) boost your chance of suffering genital ulcers.

causes

The most prevalent cause is STIs. Ulcers in the genital region may arise if you have:

- Chancroid, which is a bacterial condition that creates open sores.
- Chlamydia.
- Genital herpes.
- Human immunodeficiency virus (HIV).
- Syphilis.
- Noninfectious ulcers like aphthous ulcers (like canker sores) or Behçet's illness.

Nonsexually acquired genital ulceration

Causes of genital ulcer disease not linked to STIs include:

- Viruses
- Cytomegalovirus, which causes viral hepatitis, encephalitis and more.
- Epstein-Barr, which causes mononucleosis (mono).
- Influenza A, which causes the flu.
- Paratyphoid, which causes typhoid fever.
- Varicella zoster, which causes chickenpox and shingles.
- Bacteria Group A Streptococcus.
- Mycoplasma pneumoniae.
- Certain medical diseases, particularly ones that produce long-term inflammation
- Behçet's disease.

- Bullous pemphigoid.
- Contact dermatitis.
- Crohn's disease.
- Cyclic neutropenia.
- Erosive lichen planus.
- Pemphigus.
- Vaginal yeast infections.
- Vulvar cancer.
- Trauma
- Sexual injury, when forceful sex or foreign objects (like sex toys) tear surface tissue.
- Chemical burns caused to a response to lotion, hair removal cream or skincare products.
- Constant rubbing, such as underwear that are overly tight.

How genital ulcers look like

In early stages, ulcers in your genital region may seem like tiny lumps or a rash. You may also notice enlarged lymph nodes in your groin. Ulcers progress over time, resulting in tiny breaches in surface tissue. They may also exude pus or fluid.

What do ulcers in the vaginal region feel like?
Some genital sores create no symptoms. Others are painful and make it tough to go about your regular life. You may experience:

- Burning feeling.
- Fever.
- Itchy genitals.
- Painful urination or sexual intercourse.
- Vaginal discharge that may smell terrible.

Diagnosis and Tests

Since genital ulcer illness has so many causes, it's necessary to obtain a complete assessment. Your healthcare professional will start by knowing more about your medical history and lifestyle. They may question you about sexual activities to identify STI risk.

The examination will involve a physical exam. Your healthcare practitioner will check at the ulcers and adjacent skin. They may also check other parts of your pelvis, such as the lymph nodes in your groin.

You may require lab testing to discover the source of the ulcers. These may include:

- Biopsy. Blood test.
- Urinalysis.

Management and Treatment

The therapy that's best for you depends on the reason. Many individuals feel better with drugs that help the body remove viruses and illnesses. These include antibiotics for bacterial illnesses or antiviral medicines for viral infections. Genital ulcer therapy may also involve ointment you apply to the wounds to encourage healing.

For genital ulcers not caused by STIs, it may benefit to consult a specialist for additional assessment. A dermatologist can diagnose the source of skin lesions. You may need to consult an infectious disease specialist for ulcers linked to uncommon viruses. This physician can also undertake sophisticated testing for ulcers that don't respond to traditional treatments.

Prevention

There are things you may do to avoid some causes of genital ulcers. These include:

- Avoid tight-fitting pants or undergarments.
- Limit closeness to one person. That individual should only be intimate with you as well.
- Practice safe sex by wearing a condom or dental dam every time.
- Stay on top of therapy for persistent disorders that might lead to genital ulcers.

- Wash your genital region everyday with mild soap.

Prognosis

If you obtain the right treatments, genital ulcer treatment is typically effective. It can take a few days for you to feel better. Most individuals make a complete recovery.

If symptoms don't improve, the treatment you are practicing may not be the proper one. Additional tests may decide which therapy you require. It's also crucial to understand that genital ulcers might come back following therapy. If you have unprotected intercourse, you may get another STI, putting you at risk for subsequent ulcers.

Self-care methods often provide quick relief. These include:

- **Warm compress for itching or pain :** Soak a hand towel in warm water. Wring it out before applying to your skin with mild pressure.
- **Cool compress for swelling:** This therapy is like a warm compress but with cool water.
- **Sitz bath for general discomfort:** Fill a bathtub with enough water so it covers your hips when you sit in it. Warm but not hot water may feel nicest. Soak a few times a day for at least 15-30 minutes.

Foods that may help treat genital ulcers

Some foods may aid with the healing of genital ulcers by lowering inflammation, combating infection, and stimulating tissue repair. These foods include:

1- Probiotics: These are live creatures that may help balance the bacteria in the digestive system and the genitals. They may also help lower the quantity of dangerous germs that cause ulcers, speed up the healing process, and alleviate certain symptoms. Probiotics may be found in fermented foods including yogurt, kefir, sauerkraut, miso, and kimchi. You can take them as supplements.

2- Colorful fruits: These fruits include substances called flavonoids, which are antioxidants that may protect the cells from harm and inflammation. Flavonoids may also help prevent or cure ulcers produced by H. pylori bacterium, one of the most prevalent causes of peptic ulcers. Some fruits high in flavonoids include blueberries, raspberries, strawberries, elderberries, blackberries, and black olives.

3- Whole grains: These grains are abundant in fiber, which may aid with digestion and avoid constipation. Constipation may increase the symptoms of ulcers by raising pressure and discomfort in the belly and the genitals. Whole grains also include vitamins and minerals that are vital for wound healing and immunological function. Some examples of whole grains include oats, barley, quinoa, buckwheat, and brown rice.

4- Lean meats, fish, eggs, and soy: These foods are rich sources of protein, which is the building block of tissues and cells. Protein is important for the healing and regeneration of the skin and the mucous membranes that border the genitals. Protein also helps combat infection and inflammation by strengthening the immune system. Some lean foods are skinless chicken and lean beef. Some fish high in omega-3 fatty acids, which have anti-inflammatory qualities, include salmon, tuna, mackerel, and sardines. Eggs and soy products like tofu and tempeh are also rich in protein.

5- Healthy fats: These fats may help lubricate and protect the skin and the mucous membranes from additional damage and irritation. They may also decrease inflammation and enhance blood flow to the afflicted regions. Some good fats include olive oil, avocado oil, nuts, and seeds.

Diets

Based on the foods that may assist with the healing of genital ulcers, I have picked some recipes that are simple to make and healthy. These dishes include:

1- Yogurt parfait: A yogurt parfait is a tasty and healthful breakfast or dessert that consists of layers of yogurt, granola, and fruit.
- Mix together yogurt, maple syrup, and vanilla in a medium bowl.
- Combine strawberries and blueberries in a small bowl.
- Place ¼ cup yogurt in a transparent glass. You now top with ¼ cup granola, and then, ¼ cup berries.
- Repeat layers one more time.
- Serve parfaits immediately or refrigerate until you are ready to eat.
- Enjoy your yogurt parfait! You may also add some honey, almonds, chocolate chips, or other toppings for more taste and crunch.

2- Oatmeal with honey and nuts:
- Add the oats to water or milk in a saucepan. Bring to a boil over high heat. Reduce the heat to medium and simmer for 5 minutes, or until the oats are cooked through.
- Stir in the honey, butter, and cinnamon (if using). You may vary the quantity of honey and butter according to your taste.

- Sprinkle the nuts on top of the porridge. You may use whatever mix of nuts you choose, such as pecans, almonds, hazelnuts, or macadamia nuts.
- Enjoy your oatmeal with honey and nuts! You may also add some fresh or dried fruits for more taste and nutrition.

3- Salmon with quinoa and broccoli: OK, I can make a note on how to prepare salmon with quinoa and broccoli, based on some online search results:
- To cook salmon with quinoa and broccoli, you will need the following ingredients: salmon fillets, quinoa, broccoli, olive oil, lime juice, salt, pepper, and any additional ingredients you choose.
- Preheat a grill pan over medium-high heat. Season the salmon fillets with salt, pepper, and any other ingredients you want. Grill for approximately 10 minutes on each side or until the salmon is cooked to your preference.
-You now rinse the quinoa in a fine-mesh strainer under cold water. Transfer to a medium saucepan and add water according to the package guidelines. Bring to a boil, then decrease the heat and simmer until the quinoa is fluffy and the water is absorbed, approximately 15 to 20 minutes.
- Cut the broccoli into tiny florets and steam them in a steamer basket or over boiling water until crisp-tender, approximately 5 to 10 minutes.
- You now prepare the dressing by whisking together the olive oil, salt, lime juice and pepper in a small bowl.

- To serve, divide the cooked quinoa among four dishes. Top with the grilled salmon and steamed broccoli. Drizzle with the dressing and enjoy your healthy and wonderful dinner

4- Chicken and vegetable soup:

To prepare chicken and vegetable soup, you will need the following ingredients: vegetable oil, skinless boneless chicken breasts, onion, garlic, chicken broth, red potatoes, cabbage, carrot, eggs (optional), salt, pepper, and any herbs or spices you choose.

- Heat vegetable oil in a big saucepan over medium heat. Add chicken breasts, onion, and garlic; cook and stir until chicken is no longer pink in the middle, approximately 5 minutes.

- Pour chicken broth into the saucepan; come to a boil. Stir in potatoes, cabbage, and carrot. Simmer soup until potatoes are soft, 30 to 40 minutes.

- Bring soup back to a boil. Drizzle in eggs and stir until cooked, approximately 1 minute (optional). Season with salt, pepper, and any other herbs or spices you want.

5- Tofu and vegetable stir-fry:

- Cut a block of extra-firm tofu into half-inch cubes and press them with a paper towel to remove excess water.

- Season the tofu with soy sauce and cornstarch and toss to coat.

- Heat some oil in a big pan or wok over high heat and cook the tofu for approximately 10 minutes, flipping regularly, until golden and crisp.
- Transfer the tofu to a platter and keep it heated.
- In the same pan, add extra oil and stir-fry your choice of veggies, such as broccoli, bell pepper, carrot, bok choy, mushroom, or bean sprouts, for approximately 6 minutes, until crisp-tender.
- Add some minced garlic and ginger and simmer for another minute, stirring regularly.
- In a small bowl, stir together some soy sauce, vegetable broth, honey, and sesame oil and pour over the veggies. Bring to a boil and simmer until slightly thickened, stirring periodically.
- Return the tofu to the pan and stir to mix with the sauce and veggies.
- Serve hot with rice or noodles, if preferred.

6- Smoothie with kefir, banana, and turmeric: Kefir is a fermented milk drink that includes probiotics, which are helpful for your gut health and digestion. Banana provides natural sweetness and potassium, which helps regulate blood pressure and muscular function. Turmeric is a spice that contains anti-inflammatory and antioxidant qualities, due to its main component curcumin. It also gives the smoothie a golden tint and a pleasant taste.

To create this smoothie, you will need the following ingredients:

- 1 cup of plain or vanilla kefir
- 1 ripe banana, peeled and sliced
- 1/4 teaspoon of powdered turmeric - A dash of black pepper (optional, but helps enhance the absorption of curcumin)
- Honey or maple syrup for it to taste (optional)

To create this smoothie, follow these steps:

- Add all the ingredients to a blender and mix until smooth and frothy. You may add some ice cubes if you like a cooler drink.
- Pour the smoothie into a glass and enjoy. You may sprinkle it with some shredded coconut or chopped almonds if you prefer.

Stomach ulcers

A stomach ulcer, sometimes termed a gastric ulcer, is an open sore that forms in the stomach lining. You may also acquire one in your duodenum, the initial section of the small intestine that your stomach feeds into. Duodenal ulcers and stomach ulcers are both kinds of peptic ulcers. They're called after pepsin, one of the digestive liquids that are present in the stomach and that can seep into the duodenum. These juices are a contributing in peptic ulcer disease.

Peptic ulcers arise when the protective mucous lining of your stomach and duodenum has been damaged, enabling gastric acids and digestive enzymes to eat away at your stomach and duodenal walls. This ultimately leads to open sores that are repeatedly inflamed by the acid. If left untreated, they might begin to create major consequences, such as internal bleeding. Over time, they may even wear a hole all the way through. This is a medical emergency.

How prevalent are stomach ulcers?

Stomach ulcers are fairly prevalent in Western nations. In the United States, there are around 4 million instances every year. Some estimates claim that 1 in 10 individuals will have one at some time in their life. That's because many of the conditions that lead to stomach ulcers are ubiquitous in Western living. Fortunately, these reasons can be discovered and reversed, giving

ulcers a chance to heal and the stomach lining a chance
to recover.

Causes of stomach ulcers

The two most prevalent reasons are:

H. pylori infection.
Helicobacter pylori (H. pylori), a sneaky bacteria,
infiltrates the stomach, leaving a path of mystery in its
wake. It is the principal reason behind peptic ulcers,
gastritis, and possibly stomach cancer.
 H. pylori is a bacterium species that takes up home in
the stomach lining. Approximately 30% to 40% persons
in the United States bear this enigmatic visitor. H. pylori
infection is the major cause of peptic ulcers. It also
promotes gastritis and inflammation of the stomach
lining. In certain situations, this bacteria may contribute
to stomach cancer.

Curiously, most infected people remain symptom-free.
Some persons exhibit natural resilience to H. pylori's
damaging effects. Signs and symptoms commonly
linked to gastritis or peptic ulcers:

- Upper abdomen discomfort (dull or burning) is
  the most prevalent symptom.
- Pain intensifies when the stomach is empty.
- Nausea and Appetite Loss.

- A sensation of fullness, frequent burping, and bloating.
- Unintended Weight Loss

H. pylori spreads by direct contact with saliva, vomit, or feces.
Contaminated food or water may also host these elusive germs.
Most infections arise throughout infancy.
Crowded living areas and unstable clean water enhance danger.

Overuse of NSAIDs

Nonsteroidal anti-inflammatory medicines (NSAIDs) are pharmaceuticals that help alleviate pain, lower fever, and decrease inflammation. These medications are extensively used to treat numerous disorders that produce pain, stiffness, or inflammation. Here are some crucial aspects concerning NSAIDs:

How They Work

NSAIDs operate by inhibiting a particular set of enzymes called cyclo-oxygenase enzymes (COX enzymes).
These enzymes are involved in creating prostaglandins, which are molecules having hormone-like actions.
Prostaglandins have a part in processes such as inflammation, blood flow, and blood clot formation.

By suppressing COX enzymes, NSAIDs can relieve pain and inflammation.

NSAIDs are used to relieve mild-to-moderate pain associated with different disorders, including:
- Headaches
- Menstrual pain
- Migraines
- Osteoarthritis
- Rheumatoid arthritis
- Sprains and strains
- Toothache

Even while NSAIDs are effective pain relievers , they have their adverse effects when too much is used . One of the negative effects is peptic ulcers.
 NSAIDs interfere with the stomach's capacity to defend itself against gastric acids. Normally, the stomach contains three defensive mechanisms:
- Mucus production: Foveolar cells lining the stomach create mucus.

- Bicarbonate production: Foveolar cells release bicarbonate, which neutralizes stomach acid.

- Blood circulation: Blood flow contributes in healing and rebuilding stomach mucosal cells.

NSAIDs inhibit the synthesis of protective mucus and change its structure. These medicines also disrupt enzymes involved in making specific protective prostaglandins in the stomach lining.When prostaglandins are reduced, the mucosal layer becomes susceptible, leading to inflammation and probable ulcer development.

Over-the-counter NSAIDs for infrequent usage (like headaches) normally don't cause ulcers. However, long-term and high-dose NSAID usage (for chronic pain or inflammatory diseases) may raise the risk.

Less common causes of stomach ulcers include:

Zollinger-Ellison Syndrome

ZES is an uncommon digestive condition characterized by excessive production of stomach acid. The major cause is a form of tumor called a gastrinoma, which secretes the hormone gastrin. Gastrinomas lead to an overproduction of stomach acid, culminating in the development of peptic ulcers.

Symptoms of Zollinger-Ellison Syndrome:

- Abdominal pain and diarrhea are frequent symptoms.
- Chronic diarrhea (often with greasy stools).
- Pain in the esophagus, particularly after meals or during night.
- Nausea, vomiting (often with blood), and wheezing.
- Malnourishment owing to decreased nutrition absorption.
- Loss of appetite.

Gastrin usually induces parietal cells in the stomach to release acid.

In ZES, gastrinomas disturb this control, resulting in excessive acid production.

The increased acidity leads to the production of peptic ulcers in the stomach, duodenum, and infrequently the jejunum.

Gastritis

Gastritis is an irritation , inflammation or erosion of the stomach lining . The stomach lining functions as a protective barrier that guards the stomach wall. When this lining weakens or receives injury, digestive fluids may harm and inflame it. Several factors may raise the risk of gastritis, including:

1. Infection: Most typically, gastritis develops from infection with the bacteria H. pylori, which is also related with stomach ulcers.

2. Alcohol Use: Excessive alcohol use might lead to gastritis.

3. Medications: Regular use of some pain medicines (such as aspirin or nonsteroidal anti-inflammatory drugs) may lead to gastritis.

4. Stress: Prolonged stress might affect the stomach lining.

5. Other illnesses: Gastritis may also arise owing to underlying illnesses including Crohn's disease, HIV/AIDS, bile reflux, or food allergies.

Symptoms of Gastritis:
- Nausea
- Abdominal bloating
- Abdominal discomfort
- Vomiting
- Indigestion
- Burning feeling in the stomach
- Hiccups
- Loss of appetite
- Black and tarry stools

consequences of Gastritis: If left untreated, gastritis may develop to many consequences, including:
- Anaemia
- Atrophic gastritis: Chronic inflammation may cause loss of the stomach lining and glands.
- Peptic ulcers: Ulcers may occur in the stomach lining or duodenum.
- Growths in the stomach lining: These growths might be benign or malignant (cancerous).
- Polyps: Small growths in the stomach.

Gastritis and stomach ulcers have similar symptoms and frequently go hand in hand. Gastritis may be a precursor to stomach ulcers, produced by the same circumstances that will ultimately cause ulcers, including H. pylori infection and mucous erosion. You may also have both.

Both gastritis and stomach ulcers may induce stomach discomfort, as well as symptoms of indigestion. Usually, the pain from an ulcer will seem more localized – like it's coming from one specific location. But because some ulcers are "silent," you may not feel it if you do have one.

If you experience symptoms of either gastritis or stomach ulcer, you should seek medical assistance. Gastritis may progress to ulcers if it hasn't already. It may also signal an infection or other problem that needs to be addressed. Medical tests can swiftly discover the reasons of your stomach ache.

Heartburn

Heartburn is a painful, burning feeling that often occurs in the center of the chest. Despite its name, it's not directly connected to the heart. Instead, heartburn is caused by stomach acid rising into the esophagus (the tube that delivers food from your mouth to your stomach). The esophagus passes through your chest, near to your heart.

Here are some crucial aspects concerning Heartburn:

Symptoms

- A searing ache in the chest, generally after eating.
- Pain that intensifies while laying down or leaning over.
- A bitter or acidic sensation in the tongue.

Heartburn may be an occasional symptom for many individuals.For others, it becomes a chronic condition, happening regularly.

Causes

Stomach acid reflux: When the lower esophageal sphincter (a muscle at the bottom of the esophagus) doesn't act correctly, stomach acid runs back up into the esophagus, creating heartburn.
Acid reflux may be worse while you're bent over or laying down.

Certain meals and beverages might provoke heartburn, including:

- Spicy foods
- Onions
- Citrus goods
- Tomato products (like ketchup)
- Fatty or fried meals
- Peppermint
- Chocolate
- Alcohol and carbonated drinks
- Large or fatty meals

Ulcer pain or heartburn?

Ulcer discomfort in your stomach region might feel quite similar to heartburn. It's commonly characterized as a scorching type of agony. Ulcer pain will be usually confined to the location of the ulcer, which is in the small intestine or stomach. Heartburn spans a greater region and tends to be higher into the chest. However, you might experience heartburn and ulcer discomfort at the same time.

Heartburn is mainly caused by acid reflux, which is when acid from your stomach flows back up through your esophagus. So, heartburn may start as low as your stomach, but it will also migrate higher from there. If your discomfort is higher than your breast bone, that's undoubtedly heartburn but it doesn't imply you don't have an ulcer too. Acid reflux can also be a symptom of a stomach ulcer.

Causes of stomach ulcer

Stomach ulcers are aggravated by stomach acid. Other individuals sense this discomfort more after they eat, whereas other people notice it more on an empty stomach.
 Let's investigate the common triggers:

1. Excessive Alcohol Consumption: Alcohol may irritate the gastric mucosa (lining of the stomach), making it more vulnerable to ulcer development.

2. Stress: While stress itself doesn't directly cause ulcers, it may increase symptoms and make existing ulcers worse.Chronic stress may damage the stomach's defensive systems.

3. Spicy meals: - Contrary to widespread perception, spicy meals do not immediately induce peptic ulcers. However, they might increase symptoms if you already have an ulcer.

Peptic ulcer illness may lead to various consequences if left untreated or badly managed. Let's investigate some possible complications:

1. Bleeding: As an ulcer erodes the stomach or duodenal wall, it may injure blood vessels, resulting in bleeding.
Symptoms of bleeding ulcers include:

- Feeling weak and dizzy upon standing.
- Vomiting blood (which may seem red or black).
- Passing tarry, black stools owing to blood in the stool.

Most bleeding ulcers may be treated endoscopically by cauterizing the blood artery or utilizing other procedures. Surgery may be indicated if endoscopic therapy fails.

2. Perforation: Rarely, an ulcer may cause a hole (perforation) in the stomach or duodenal wall. Bacteria and partly digested food might leak into the sterile abdominal cavity (peritoneum).
Symptoms of a perforated ulcer include abrupt, sharp, acute pain.

Immediate medical examination is vital, and surgical repair is typically required.

3. Narrowing and Obstruction: Ulcers at the end of the stomach (where the duodenum connects) may cause swelling and scarring.These ulcers may constrict or block the intestinal aperture, preventing the flow of food from the stomach to the small intestine.
Symptoms include vomiting and trouble eating.

Endoscopic balloon dilation may assist, although surgery could be necessary if dilation is unsuccessful.

4. Anaemia: Chronic bleeding from ulcers may lead to anaemia owing to decreasing red blood cell count. Anaemic persons may feel weary, weak, and have shortness of breath.

5. Infection: A perforated ulcer might invite infection in the abdominal cavity (peritonitis). Immediate medical intervention is important to avert major consequences.

6. Other Complications:
Internal bleeding needing hospitalization and blood transfusion.
Severe blood loss resulting to bloody vomit or stool
Delayed healing of ulcers.
Scar tissue growth that inhibits digestion.

How is a stomach ulcer diagnosed?
Your healthcare professional will question you about your symptoms and medical history. They will want to know whether you routinely take NAIDs or have a history of H. pylori infection. If indicators indicate an ulcer, they will want to have a peek inside your stomach and duodenum.

Tests

1- Endoscopy. An upper endoscopy check is efficient because it enables healthcare personnel to view within your digestive system and also obtain a tissue sample to evaluate in the lab. The test is done by passing a thin tube with a small camera attached down your neck and into your stomach and duodenum. You'll take medicine to numb your throat and help you relax throughout the exam. Your healthcare professional may use the endoscope to obtain a tissue sample to test for evidence of mucosal damage, anaemia, H. pylori infection or cancer. If the sample is taken, you won't feel it.

2- Imaging testing. Imaging tests to view within the stomach and small intestine include:

1- Upper GI series. An upper GI X-ray exam checks the stomach and duodenum with X-rays. It's less intrusive than an endoscopy. For the X-ray, you'll drink a chalky fluid called barium, which will cover your esophagus, stomach and duodenum. The barium helps your digestive organs show up better in black and white photos.

2- CT scan. Your healthcare physician would prescribe a CT scan if they need to view your organs in greater detail. A CT scan might indicate issues such as a hole in the stomach or intestinal wall. For the exam, you'll lay on a table inside a scanning machine while X-rays are taken. You may drink or receive an injection with contrast fluid to help your organs show up better on photographs.

3- Tests for H. pylori. Your healthcare practitioner may wish to test you individually for H. pylori infection. Tests may include:

4- Blood test. A blood test is a fast and straightforward approach to screen for past H. pylori infection. The lab searches for indications of antibodies to the germs in your blood. It's not as accurate for identifying an active illness, however.

5- Stool test. Healthcare practitioners may also discover H. pylori in your stool. They may want to look at your faeces if you have observed changes in it.

6- Breath test. The H. pylori breath test is a reliable test for identifying an active H. pylori infection. For the test, you'll swallow a flavored fluid containing an organic chemical molecule called urea. If H. pylori bacteria are present in your digestive system, they will break down the urea and convert it to carbon dioxide. The carbon dioxide will then come out in your breath. When you breathe into a bag, healthcare practitioners will be able to quantify it.

Management and Treatment

Ulcers may recover if they are given a respite from the circumstances that produced them. Healthcare doctors treat simple ulcers using a mix of drugs to lower stomach acid, coat and protect the ulcer during healing and eradicate any bacterial infection that may be present. Medicines may include:

1- Antibiotics. If H. pylori was detected in your digestive system, your healthcare practitioner will prescribe some combination of medicines to kill the bacterium, depending on your medical history and condition. Commonly recommended antibiotics include tetracycline, metronidazole, clarithromycin and amoxicillin.

2- Proton pump inhibitors (PPIs). These medications help lower stomach acid and preserve your stomach lining. Some of these PPIs include omeprazole , esomeprazole , lansoprazole, dexlansoprazole, rabeprazole and also pantoprazole.

3- Histamine receptor blockers (H2 blockers). These lower stomach acid by inhibiting the chemical that signals your body to create it (histamines). H2 blockers include cimetidine , nizatidine and famotidine.

4- Antacids. These common over-the-counter medicines help to neutralize stomach acid. They may deliver some symptom relief, but they aren't enough to cure your ulcer. They also could interact with certain antibiotics.

5- Cytoprotective agents. These drugs assist to cover and preserve your stomach lining. They include sucralfate and misoprostol.
Bismuth Subsalicylate. This over-the-counter drug, typically marketed as Pepto-Bismol, may help cover and protect your ulcer from stomach acid. (Note: Bismuth could color your feces black, but this effect appears different from the sticky, tarry appearance of blood in your excrement.)

Lifestyle Modifications

1- Avoid Irritants: Limit or avoid alcohol, smoke, and spicy meals.

2- Reduce Stress: Practice relaxation methods like deep breathing or meditation.

3- Dietary Changes: Consume smaller, more frequent meals. Avoid eating late at night.

4- Limit NSAIDs: If you take nonsteroidal anti-inflammatory medicines (NSAIDs), seek alternatives with your doctor.

After commencing therapy, a follow-up endoscopy may be conducted to monitor ulcer healing and check for H. pylori eradication.
If H. pylori is still present, more antibiotic therapy may be required.

Surgery (Rare)

While most ulcers are effectively managed with medicine, certain complex ulcers may need surgery. Ulcers that are bleeding, or that have perforated your stomach or intestinal wall, will need to be medically healed. An ulcer that is cancerous, or restricting a channel, will need to be surgically removed. In extreme situations, an ulcer that keeps coming back may be treated by surgery to cut off portion of the nerve supply to the stomach that creates stomach acid.Surgical alternatives include vagotomy, antrectomy, or partial gastrectomy.

Regular follow-up visits with your healthcare physician
are crucial to check progress.
Prevent recurrence by sticking to recommended drugs
and lifestyle adjustments.

How soon after therapy will I feel better?

The healing period for a stomach ulcer may vary
depending on numerous variables, including the kind of
ulcer, its severity, and the success of therapy. Here are
some broad guidelines:

1. Small, Superficial Ulcers: These may heal within a
few weeks to a couple of months with adequate
treatment. Lifestyle adjustments (such as avoiding
irritants and stress) and drugs (such proton pump
inhibitors or H2 blockers) may enhance recovery.

2. Larger or Chronic Ulcers: Chronic ulcers (those that
remain for a long time) may take many months to
heal.Treatment frequently comprises a combination of
drugs to lower acid production, eliminate H. pylori (if
present), and preserve the stomach lining.

3. H. pylori-Related Ulcers:
If the ulcer is caused by H. pylori, effective eradication of
the bacteria is vital.Antibiotic medication normally lasts
for around 1 to 2 weeks.
Follow-up endoscopy confirms healing following
therapy.

4. Individual Variability: Healing periods may vary greatly from person to person.Factors including general health, adherence to therapy, and lifestyle have a role.

Is diet needed for ulcer healing?

While healing from a stomach ulcer, nutrition plays a significant role in promoting recovery and minimizing aggravation. Here are some dietary recommendations:

1. Soft and Bland meals: Opt for meals that are easy on the stomach. These include: Cooked cereals (such as oatmeal or cream of wheat).
- Rice.
- Mashed potatoes.
- Boiled eggs.
- Cooked veggies (avoid spicy or sour ones).
- Bananas (which are simple to digest).

2. Avoid Irritants:
- Spicy meals, citrus fruits, and tomato-based products may increase ulcer symptoms.
- Limit caffeine (from coffee, tea, and chocolate) and alcohol.

3. Small, Frequent Meals:
- Instead of huge meals, take smaller quantities more frequently.

- This helps minimize stomach acid production and avoids overwhelming the digestive system.

4. Protein Sources:
- Include lean proteins such as:
- Chicken, turkey , or fish.
- Tofu.
- Eggs.

5. Healthy Fats:
- Opt for healthy fats like those found in avocado, olive oil, and almonds.
   - Avoid fried or oily meals.

6. Dairy Products:
- Some individuals receive relief from ulcers by ingesting milk, yoghurt, or kefir. However, if dairy worsens your symptoms, avoid it.

7. Fluids:
- Stay hydrated by drinking lots of water.
   - Herbal drinks (such as chamomile or ginger) might relieve the stomach.

8. Avoid Late-Night Eating:
- Eating close to sleep might cause acid reflux.
   - Aim to complete your last meal at least 2-3 hours before bedtime.

9. Individual Tolerance:

- Pay attention to how your body reacts to various meals.
   - Keep a food journal to monitor any triggers or discomfort.

When is it an emergency?

Seek immediate attention in the ER if you suffer any of the following symptoms associated to stomach ulcers:

1. Severe Abdominal Pain:

- If you experience significant, continuous pain in your belly that doesn't lessen, it's vital to get emergency medical assistance.

2. Signs of Bleeding:

   - Bloody Stools: If you observe blood in your stools, it might suggest bleeding from an ulcer.
   - Bloody Vomit: Vomiting a material that resembles coffee grounds may also be an indication of bleeding.

3. Severe Blood Loss:

- Symptoms such as paleness, faintness, or feeling exceedingly weak might indicate severe blood loss.
- These indicators necessitate prompt investigation and treatment.

Foods that may help cure stomach ulcers

Some meals that may help treat stomach ulcers are:

1- meals rich in antioxidants: These meals may protect your stomach lining and fight against the H. pylori infection. Examples of antioxidant-rich foods include blueberries, cherries, bell peppers, broccoli, leafy greens, and olive oil.

2- Foods containing probiotics: These foods may help restore the balance of healthy bacteria in your gut and avoid reinfection. Examples of probiotic-rich foods include yogurt, kefir, miso, sauerkraut, and kombucha.

3- Meals having anti-inflammatory properties: These meals may lessen inflammation and discomfort in your stomach. Examples of anti-inflammatory foods include honey, garlic, turmeric, and licorice.

4- Meals that neutralize stomach acid: These meals may help ease the burning feeling and pain produced by excess acid in your stomach. Examples of acid-neutralizing foods include milk, bananas, oats, and rice.

Recipes

1- Cabbage soup: Cabbage is a natural ulcer cure that includes vitamin C and antioxidants, which may help

preserve your stomach lining and fight against H. pylori infection. To prepare cabbage soup, you will need:
- 1/4 head of cabbage, chopped
- 2 carrots, peeled and sliced
- 1 onion, diced
- 2 cloves of garlic, minced
- 4 cups of vegetable broth
- Salt and pepper to taste
- Parsley for garnish
 - In a large saucepan, heat some oil over medium-high heat and sauté the onion and garlic until tender, approximately 10 minutes. Add the cabbage and carrots and simmer for another 10 minutes, stirring regularly. Add the broth and bring to a boil. Reduce the heat and simmer until the cabbage and carrots are soft, approximately 20 minutes. You then season with salt and pepper and sprinkle with parsley and you are good to go.

2- Banana smoothie: Bananas are a wonderful source of potassium, fiber, and vitamin B6, which may help cure stomach ulcers by neutralizing stomach acid and improving the mucous layer. To prepare a banana smoothie, you will need:
- 2 ripe bananas, peeled and sliced
- 1 cup of plain yogurt or you can use kefir
- 1/4 cup of milk or almond milk
- 1 spoonful of honey
- A teaspoon of cinnamon

- In a blender, add all the ingredients and blend until smooth and creamy. Pour into a glass and you are good to go.

3- Honey garlic chicken: Honey and garlic are both foods with anti-inflammatory characteristics that may help relieve discomfort and inflammation in your stomach. To prepare honey garlic chicken, you will need:
- 4 chicken breasts, boneless and skinless
- 1/4 cup of honey
- 2 teaspoons of soy sauce
- 4 cloves of garlic, minced
- Salt and pepper to taste
- In a small bowl, whisk together the honey, soy sauce, and garlic. Season the chicken with salt and pepper and put in a baking dish. Pour the honey garlic sauce over the chicken and bake in a preheated oven at 375°F (190°C) for 25 to 30 minutes, or until the chicken is cooked through and the sauce is bubbling. Serve with rice or steaming veggies.

4- Turmeric rice: Turmeric is a spice that has been demonstrated to have anti-ulcer and anti-H. pylori properties in animal and human tests. To prepare turmeric rice, you will need:
- 1 cup of basmati rice, washed and drained
- 2 cups of water
- 1 teaspoon of turmeric
- 1/4 teaspoon of salt
- 2 teaspoons of butter

- In a medium saucepan, bring the water to a boil and add the rice, turmeric, and salt. Stir thoroughly and decrease the heat to low. Cover and cook until the rice is soft and the water is absorbed, approximately 15 to 20 minutes. Fluff with a fork and whisk in the butter. Serve hot or cold.

5- Blueberry muffins: Blueberries are rich in antioxidants and flavonoids, which may help prevent and cure H. pylori infection and stomach ulcers . To make blueberry muffins, you will need the following:
 - 2 cups of all-purpose flour
- 2 tablespoons of baking powder
- 1/2 teaspoon of salt
- 1/4 cup of sugar
- 1/4 cup of oil
- 1 egg, beaten
- 3/4 cup of milk
- 1 cup of frozen or fresh blueberries
- In a bowl, mix together the flour, baking powder, sugar and salt . In a small bowl, mix together the oil, milk, and egg . You then add the wet ingredients to the dry ones and whisk until just incorporated. Gently fold in the blueberries. Now spoon the batter into a prepared muffin tray and bake in a preheated oven at 375°F (190°C) for 18 to 20 minutes, or until brown and a toothpick inserted comes out clean. Cool on a wire rack and enjoy!

6- Oatmeal with milk: Oatmeal is a relaxing and nourishing diet that may help cure stomach ulcers by covering the stomach lining and lowering acid

production . Milk is also a food that may help neutralize gastric acid and offer calcium and protein. To cook oatmeal with milk, you will need:
 - 1/2 cup of rolled oats
- 1 cup of milk or almond milk
- A teaspoon of salt
- In a small saucepan, bring the milk and salt to a boil and add the oats. Reduce the heat and simmer, stirring periodically, until the oats are soft and creamy, approximately 10 to 15 minutes. You may also add some honey, cinnamon, or fruits for added taste and nutrients.

9 798883 066602